A Workshop Approach
to Arthur Miller's

Death of a Salesman

Kopiervorlagen
von Brenda Pinder

Ernst Klett Schulbuchverlag
Stuttgart Düsseldorf Berlin Leipzig

A Workshop Approach to Arthur Miller's Death of a Salesman

Kopiervorlagen von Brenda Pinder

Contents

Bildnachweis
Archiv für Kunst und Geschichte, Berlin: Umschlagfoto (Erich Ponto als Willy, 1950); Deutsches Theatermuseum, München, Archiv Heinz Köster: S. 19; International Correspondence Schools, Scranton, Pa.: S. 6, 10; Kinoarchiv Engelmeier, Hamburg: S. 9, 20; Dumont-Lindemann-Archiv Düsseldorf: S. 11. Nicht in allen Fällen war es uns möglich, den uns bekannten Rechteinhaber der Abbildungen ausfindig zu machen. Berechtigte Ansprüche werden selbstverständlich im Rahmen der üblichen Vereinbarungen abgegolten.

1. Auflage 1 5 4 3 2 | 1997 96 95 94

Alle Drucke dieser Auflage können im Unterricht nebeneinander benutzt werden, sie sind untereinander unverändert. Die letzte Zahl bezeichnet das Jahr dieses Druckes.

Satz: Setzerei Lihs, Ludwigsburg
Druck: Gutmann + Co GmbH, Heilbronn
ISBN 3-12-577631-7

Preface

The activities in this book are inspired by a conviction that students learn a good deal more about drama texts if they are encouraged to treat them first and foremost as plays – as scripts that are not complete without performance of some kind – and that active participation in their own learning process is essential to real understanding. So the activities are intended to help students explore the play for themselves, with the teacher as guide, rather than be told about it by critics or "experts". Nevertheless the teacher remains indispensible, since help and guidance are needed. The teacher, too, may gain new insights through this shared exploration.

Teachers do not need to be experienced or trained in drama teaching to use these copy masters. All exercises are fully explained and not at all threatening – neither to teachers, nor to students!

The activities fall into two sections. Part A is meant to lead into the play by introducing important themes and approaches to stagecraft *before* the whole play is read. An understanding of the way Miller balances past and present, for instance, and the concepts of success and the American Dream, seem necessary preliminaries to a full reading.

Part B, which helps students to find a way through plot and structure, character, themes and technical devices, may be used in any order (the one offered is only a suggestion, and the strategies may either be sandwiched between close readings of the text or may follow it.

References throughout are to the Klett edition of *Death of a Salesman* (KLETTBUCH 57763) but can be easily adapted to any other edition.

My thanks are due to colleagues and tutors on the *Shakespeare and Schools Project* of the Cambridge Institute of Education for many of the "active approaches" which I have adapted to use on this play, and for their reinforcement of my belief that plays are *scripts* rather than "texts".

Brenda Pinder

PART A Preliminary Exercises

Units 1 to 5 introduce students to the setting of the play before they read it. They are also led to think about some aspects of plot and structure. This is done creatively: students get involved in Willy's world, questioning the American Dream and its manifestation in the world of business. Secondly, students catch a glimpse of Miller's world, the stage, by experimenting with set design and the dramatic portrayal of past and present side by side.

Impulse

Read through the following statements with a partner.

1. "What I want most out of life is plenty of money so that I can buy whatever I and my family need."
2. "I value the good opinion of my friends and family more than money; I want respect and popularity."
3. "I need to be able to say at the end of my life that I have achieved something worthwhile."
4. "Happiness comes through serving other people rather than being selfish."
5. "Providing well for my family is very important to me; I want to give my children a good start in life."
6. "Education is vital to the quality of life."

Activity

Discuss each of these statements with your partner and see if you can agree on their order of importance.
Look at the statements you each ranked highly. What do they tell you about yourselves?
When you make your own choice, to what extent are you influenced by the values of your parents and of the society you live in?

Use this exchange of ideas with your partner as preparation for a class discussion on the following issues:

The values of our present society
and
How do we define success?

Follow-up

Now read these lines drawn from the play you are about to study.

a) ". . . it's what I always wanted. My own apartment, a car, and plenty of women."

b) ". . . the man who makes an appearance in the business world, the man who creates personal interest, is the man who gets ahead. Be liked and you will never want."

c) "To suffer fifty weeks of the year for the sake of a two-week vacation, when all you really desire is to be outdoors, with your shirt off. And always to have to get ahead of the next fella."

d) "It's not what you do, Ben. It's who you know and the smile on your face!"

e) "The only thing you got in this world is what you can sell."

f) "Never fight fair with a stranger, boy. You'll never get out of the jungle that way."

Again, working in pairs, discuss what attitudes to life are reflected in these statements, and what view of success.

Look at the advertisement from the 1920s (next page), the time in which Willy Loman would have been starting his career. Pick out statements that resemble some of the above quotes from the play. Are there any marked differences?

Try to sum up the ideas you have discussed in a few brief notes; you will find them very useful later.

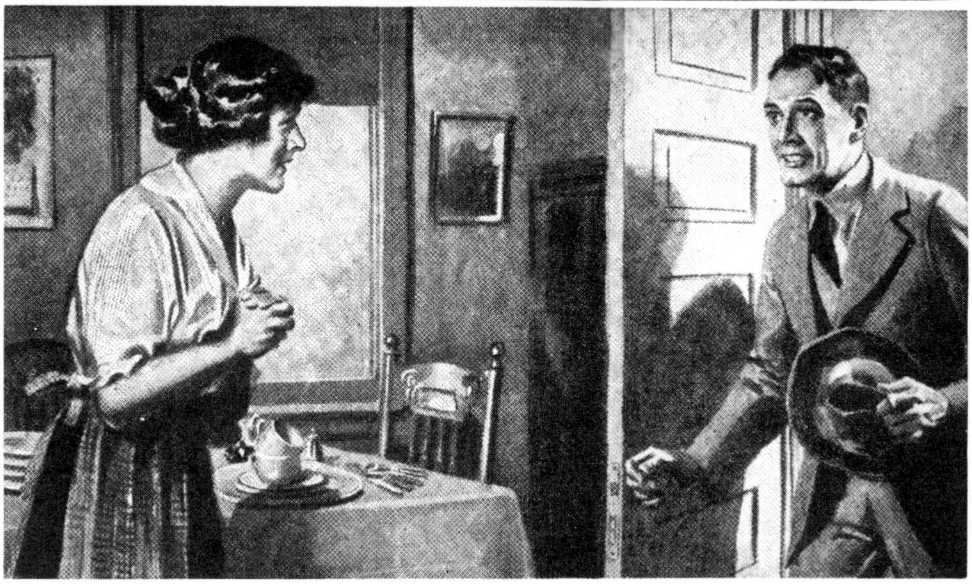

"I Got the Job!"

"I'm to be Manager of my Department starting Monday. The boss said he had been watching all the men. When he found I had been studying at home with the International Correspondence Schools he knew I had the right stuff in me—that I was bound to make good. Now we can move over to that house on Oakland Avenue and you can have a maid and take things easy. I tell you, Nell, taking that course with the I. C. S. was the best thing I ever did."

Spare-time study with the I. C. S. is winning promotions for thousands of men and bringing happiness to thousands of homes all over the world. In offices, shops, stores, mines, mills and on railroads, I. C. S. trained men are stepping up to big jobs, over the heads of older men, past those whose only qualification is long service.

There is a job ahead of *you* that some man is going to be picked for. The boss can't take chances. When he selects the one to hold it he is going to choose a trained man with sound, practical knowledge of the work. Get busy right now and put yourself in line for that promotion. You can do it in spare time in your own home through the International Correspondence Schools, just as nearly two million men have done in the last twenty-five years, just as more than 100,000 men are doing today.

The first step these men took was to mark and mail this coupon. Make *your* start the same way—and make it right now.

INTERNATIONAL CORRESPONDENCE SCHOOLS
Scranton, Pa. Montreal, Can.

TEAR OUT HERE

INTERNATIONAL CORRESPONDENCE SCHOOLS
BOX 2168, SCRANTON, PA.

Explain, without obligating me, how I can qualify for the position, or in the subject, *before* which I mark X.

- ☐ ELECTRICAL ENGINEER
- ☐ Electric Lighting and Railways
- ☐ Electric Wiring
- ☐ Telegraph Engineer
- ☐ Telephone Work
- ☐ MECHANICAL ENGINEER
- ☐ Mechanical Draftsman
- ☐ Machine Shop Practice
- ☐ Gas Engine Operating
- ☐ CIVIL ENGINEER
- ☐ Surveying and Mapping
- ☐ MINE FOREMAN OR ENGINEER
- ☐ Metallurgist or Prospector
- ☐ STATIONARY ENGINEER
- ☐ Marine Engineer
- ☐ Ship Draftsman
- ☐ ARCHITECT
- ☐ Contractor and Builder
- ☐ Architectural Draftsman
- ☐ Concrete Builder
- ☐ Structural Engineer
- ☐ PLUMBING AND HEATING
- ☐ Sheet Metal Worker
- ☐ Textile Overseer or Supt.
- ☐ CHEMIST
- ☐ SALESMANSHIP
- ☐ ADVERTISING
- ☐ Window Trimmer
- ☐ Show Card Writer
- ☐ Sign Painter
- ☐ Railroad Trainman
- ☐ ILLUSTRATING
- ☐ Cartooning
- ☐ BOOKKEEPER
- ☐ Stenographer and Typist
- ☐ Cert. Public Accountant
- ☐ TRAFFIC MANAGER
- ☐ Railway Accountant
- ☐ Commercial Law
- ☐ GOOD ENGLISH
- ☐ Teacher
- ☐ Common School Subjects
- ☐ Mathematics
- ☐ CIVIL SERVICE
- ☐ Railway Mail Clerk
- ☐ AUTOMOBILE OPERATING
- ☐ Auto Repairing
- ☐ Navigation
- ☐ AGRICULTURE
- ☐ Poultry Raising
- ☐ Spanish
- ☐ French
- ☐ Italian

Name ______________________

Present Occupation ______________________

Street and No. ______________________

City __________ ______________________ **State** __________

Canadians may send this coupon to International Correspondence Schools, Montreal, Can.

Impulse

THE SALESMAN ETHIC

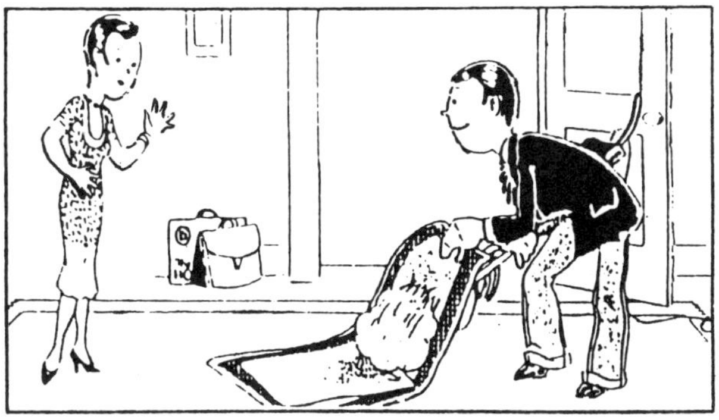

"This positive agitation test reveals dirt you never knew you had"

"Do you remember how you felt during Convention week?" asks T. H. Home, the author of a review of the 1938 Hoover European Convention in Rustington. The salesmen gathered and according to Mr. Home felt "REJUVENATED ... RE-BORN ... RE-ENTHUSED! YOU CAPTURED THE MAGIC OF HOOVER LIMITED IN YOU HEART".

Their slogans roused the passions of every salesman, an anthem of confidence, enthusiasm and opportunity:

RUSTINGTON SLOGANS

1. That we may better serve.
2. IT ALL DEPENDS ON ME.
3. Every man is my Superior in some phase of life, and in that will I learn from him.
4. It's what you DO with what you KNOW that counts.
5. Light your TORCH OF ENTHUSIASM here and KEEP IT KINDLED.
6. Make FRIENDS . . . Make MERRY . . . make THE MOST OF YOUR OPPORTUNITIES.
7. If you want to pick faults, start with YOURSELF.
8. CONFIDENCE in YOURSELF is the first step on the ROAD TO SUCCESS.
9. This is the HOOVER FILLING STATION on the ROAD TO SUCCESS.
10. The STOREHOUSE OF HOOVER KNOWLEDGE.
11. Let's INCREASE HIS EARNINGS.
12. If at first you don't succeed, TRY, TRY – TRY AGAIN.

"WE ARE THE INVINCIBLE NORTH"

Amongst the resolves and decisions of the salesman were the following:

RUSTINGTON DECISIONS
(General)

1. We will accept responsibility to impart to our men EXTRA KNOWLEDGE, CONFIDENCE, UNDER-STANDING, EXAMPLE and pledge help to INCREASE HIS EARNINGS.
2. We will master DRILL TRAINING.
3. We will give MORE STUDY to all phases of our job.
4. Our ACHIEVEMENTS will match up to our INCREASED KNOWLEDGE.
5. We will considerably improve our present efforts of A SALE FIRST WEEK FOR THE NEW MAN.
6. We will extend and encourage MORE CONTACT and CO-OPERATION with our SERVICE COLLEAGUES.
7. We will impart ALL THAT WE HAVE LEARNED AND SEEN TO OUR BROTHER SALESMAN.
8. We will insist on MORE CONSTRUCTIVE NIGHT WORK, and LEAD BY EXAMPLE.
9. We realise the answer is "NO" until she KNOWS.
10. We will generate the correct way to support "SELL IN ROTATION" plan.
11. We will insist on DAWN PATROLS, A.M. and P.M. PA-RADES, DRILL TRAINING SESSIONS, as per exposi-tion by the Sales Educational Department "HOW IT SHOULD BE DONE".
12. We will maintain ENTHUSIASM GENERATED AT CONVENTION, and BRING GREAT HONOUR TO THE GLORIOUS NORTH.

"WE WILL BE MEN OF OUR WORD"!

The accompanying leaflet is part of a training scheme used to prepare salesmen of HOOVER vacuum cleaners in the 1930s in the USA. Look especially at the Rustington slogans. (Rustington was the site of Hoover's Sales Convention in 1938.) Notice the emphasis on confidence and popularity.

Now turn to the study aids accompanying your edition of the play, pp. 119–120, "Success, Happiness and the American Dream", Section 7. (Students using another edition of the play should go on to the next step, the *Timebends* quote.) How, according to Gorer, is success measured in American society? (Remember that this is 1948, just a few months before the play was published.) Compare these ideas with the Rustington slogans. Then consider the following: In his autobiography, *Timebends,* Arthur Miller describes an incident that occurred on the opening night of *Death of a Salesman.* An outraged woman accused the play of being "a time bomb under American capitalism". That, said Miller, was what he intended – to place a "time bomb" under

"the bullshit of capitalism, this pseudo-life that thought to touch the clouds by standing on top of a refrigerator, waving a paid up mortgage at the moon, victorious at last." *(Timebends, p. 184).*

Why do you think Miller is so critical?

Activity

Imagine you are one of the Hoover salesmen in the 1930s, when vacuum cleaners were relatively new. Working with a partner, make up a dialogue with a potential customer, following the advice given. It will help if you read the tips given in Section 8 (pp. 120–121 of your edition) first. Try out your dialogue, working in improvements, details of gestures etc. You may have time to perform the scene in class.

With your partner – and perhaps with others – discuss what values and aspects of the American Dream your dialogue reflects.

Follow-up

The central character, Willy Loman, does not sell vacuum cleaners. It is never made quite clear what he *does* sell, but it is likely to be stockings and underwear. Whatever it is, he *has* absorbed the salesman principles of his society. If you look back at the statements in Unit 1, you will see that statements b) und d) reflect these values very clearly – and they are both made by him. A great deal of his energy in the play is devoted to being "well liked".

Now read through the speech that Willy Loman makes to his boss, Howard (Act II, pp. 57–58, from "I thought I'd go out" to "for months after that"). Discuss with your partner what it shows us about Willy's picture of an ideal salesman. It is really quite unlikely to be an accurate picture, but rather an idealised memory existing only in Willy's mind. Make a few more notes on this speech, as we shall be returning to it when you have finished reading through the play.

Impulse

Read the scene of conflict between Willy and Biff towards the end of the play, Act II, p. 95 l. 61 ("The man don't know who we are!") to p. 97 l. 36 ("I am Willy Loman, and you are Biff Loman!"). Then read the extract aloud in pairs, omitting Happy's and Linda's lines for the moment. The scene is the climax of a continuous conflict between Willy and his son, Biff. You will see that it clearly highlights the different views of success and morality each holds.

Activity

Divide the class into two groups, one to be Biff and the other Willy. Each student should choose **one** line from the dialogue which seems to sum up the attitude to life that the given character holds. Line up in two rows, facing one another. In turn, with Biff and Willy alternately, shout your line at the person opposite you. It doesn't matter if more than one person has chosen the same line; what you are doing is tuning in to the animosity which exists between them. Other reasons for this will become apparent in the play, but concentrate here on their views of success and what each wants from life.

Follow-up

In Act I, Willy's wife Linda makes a speech which highlights Willy's relationship to his sons from her point of view. She defends Willy against criticism, strengthening the audience's sympathy for Willy: p. 40 l. 15 ("Are they any worse than his sons?") – l. 30 (". . . a philandering bum . . .").
The teacher or a student should write each sentence of the speech on a separate card. The cards should be distributed among class members. The aim is to explore this speech for yourselves – to "walk about inside the lines". Your are to become Linda's thoughts and to deliver your section of her speech with as much feeling as you can.

Take a few minutes to discuss the language of the speech afterwards: it is essentially simple but full of feeling.

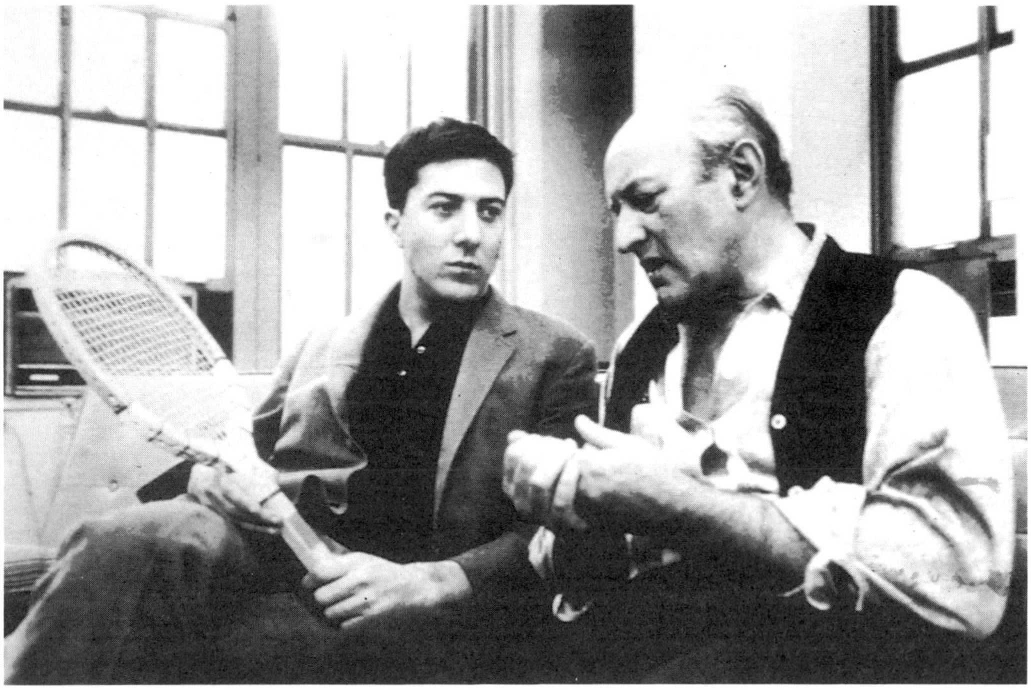

Dustin Hoffman as Bernard (left) and Lee J. Cobb as Willy, in an early theatre performance of Death of a Salesman *in New York*

Impulse

1. A young business man has the difficult task of telling an elderly employee, who has worked for the firm all his working life, that he is no longer needed and is to be made redundant.
2. The employee remembers, as he listens to the excuses and apologies, several events from earlier, happier times.

The ambitious tone of the advertisement below might give you some ideas.

Activity

First of all, work in pairs to improvise the dialogue of 1. Think how the boss would introduce the topic, and how the employee would react.

Now join with another pair to form a group of four. Decide between you on two or three of the "memories" in 2. He might remember, for instance, his first day at work, or his first pay day and what he bought for his wife and children with his money, or the day he concluded an important deal for the firm and was congratulated by the former boss . . .

Your task is to weave these memories into the first improvisation. The dialogue stops and the boss "freezes" while the employee reenacts the incident from the past with the help of other characters.

It doesn't matter what these memories show; the purpose of the activity is to give you some insight into one way of presenting past and present in the same scene.

Follow-up

Death of a Salesman is a similar, but of course more complex, mixture of past and present. One more important factor in the scenes of memory is that they are all seen through the eyes of one character – Willy Loman – and therefore reflect *his* view of past events, which may well be distorted.

Still in groups of four, think back over your improvised scenes. Do you think the past was coloured by the employee's viewpoint? Would any other character involved have given a different version? Choose one other character who appeared in the memories. One of you then adapts the role of this character and describes the incident from his or her point of view.

HERE is your future charted for you, based on the actual average earnings of trained and untrained men.

Which way will you go? You'll either go *up*, through *training*, to a position that means good money and more comforts as the years go by, or you'll go *down*, through *lack* of training, into the ranks of the poorly paid.

It rests entirely with you which way you go. You can make or break your own future. And *now* is the time to decide. Not next year, not next month, but *now*. You *can* go up if you want to. You can *get* the training that will command a trained man's salary. The International Correspondence Schools have helped hundreds of thousands of men to qualify for advancement. Let them show *you* how *you* can prepare yourself, in your own home, for the position you want in the work you like best.

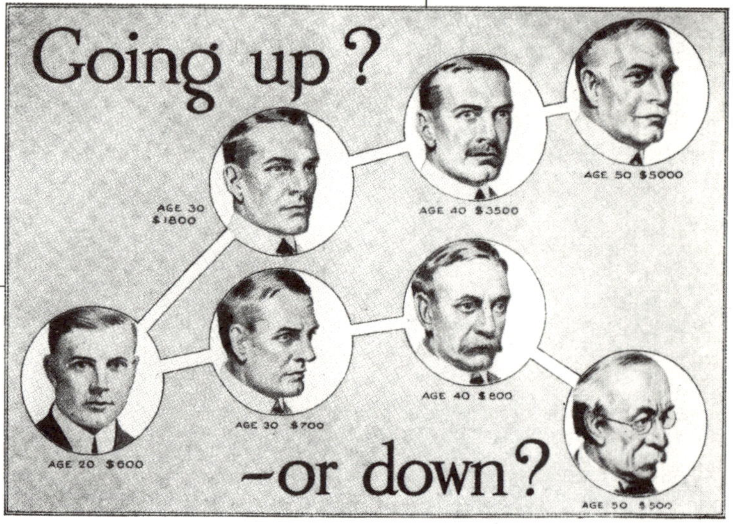
Going up?
AGE 30 $1800
AGE 40 $3500
AGE 50 $5000
AGE 20 $600
AGE 30 $700
AGE 40 $800
AGE 50 $500
–or down?

Impulse

Before you start reading the dialogue of the play, take a close look at the detailed stage directions Miller gives us about the set prior to Willy's entrance (p. 5 ll. 3 – 25).

Activity

As you will see, the setting is not just a series of instructions for the designer; there are symbolic elements, too, like the "towering angular shapes" behind the house and the "angry glow" in the lighting. Even more important are the instructions concerning the differing uses of the set in scenes of present and past.

It is therefore vital for you to have a clear idea of what Miller intends.

Work in pairs to make a stage plan of the set and a sketch of what it would look like from the auditorium. No need to be artistic – the ideas are what count, not the execution. Display your diagrams for everyone to see and discuss.

Follow-up

Now, as a class, mark out the actual setting in a suitable space, using chairs etc to set boundaries of kitchen, bedroom, yard etc. Don't just look at this from the front – from the audience's viewpoint – but walk about on the "set" you have created, to feel what the actors would experience.

This is an exercise which most directors do with their cast early on in rehearsals, so that they will see the moves in three dimensions from the start.

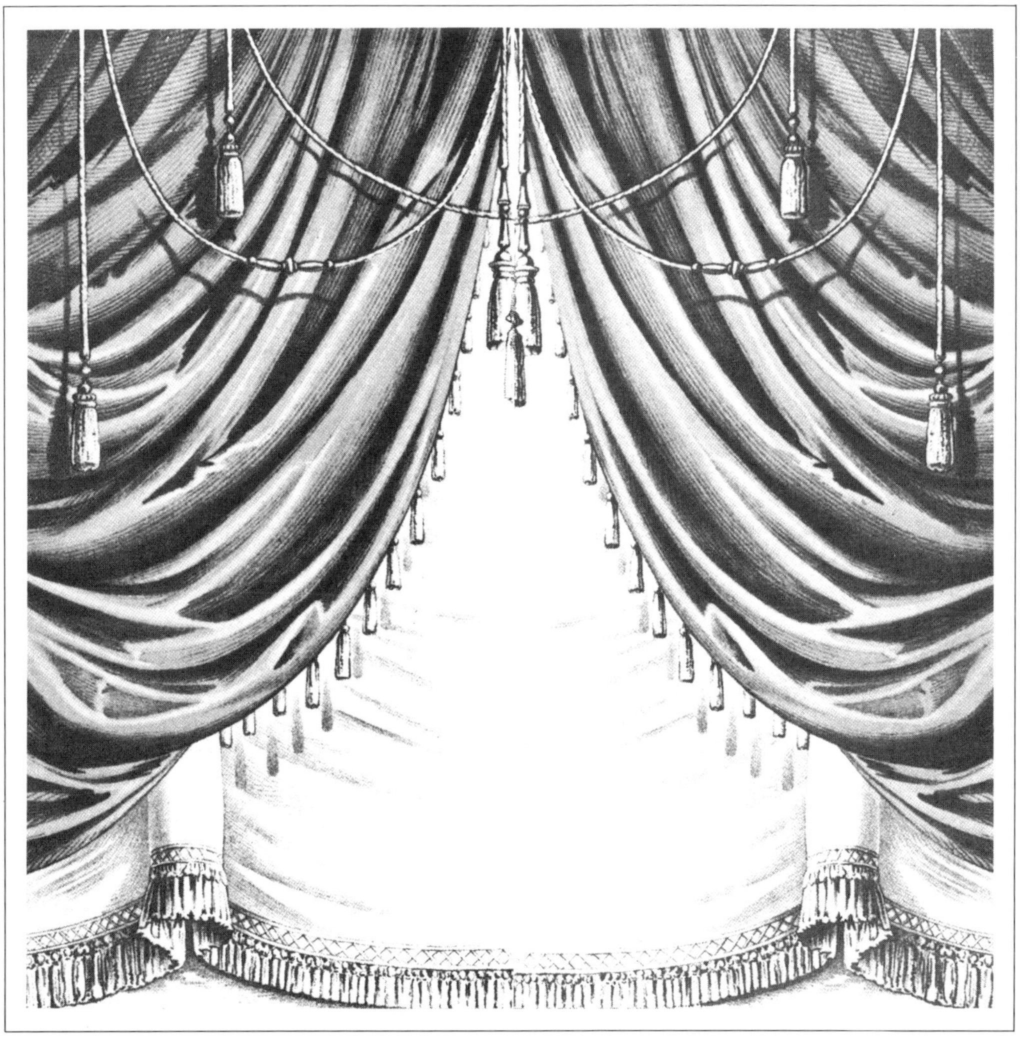

PART B Exercises on the Play

The following exercises are best undertaken parallel to, or following, a close reading of the text. Students can now apply the insights they have gained in PART A.
There is a certain degree of progression in the units of PART B, though the teacher can easily rearrange them. Since each unit is complete in itself, a change of order poses no great problems.
The exercises are varied so that the students practise oral, written and performance skills. This gives them – and the teacher – the chance to discover where their preferences and particular abilities lie. The variety of the approaches also furthers the retention of essential content and messages.

UNIT 6 Moulding a character

Impulse

Look at these three passages from the stage directions.

> *Linda, his wife, has stirred in her bed at the right. She gets out and puts on a robe, listening. Most often jovial, she has developed an iron repression of her exceptions to Willy's behavior – she more than loves him, she admires him, as though his mercurial nature, his temper, his massive dreams and little cruelties, served her only as sharp reminders of the turbulent longings within him, longings which she shares but lacks the temperament to utter and follow to their end.* (p. 6)

> *(Light has risen on the boys' room. Unseen, Willy is heard talking to himself, "eighty thousand miles," and a little laugh. Biff gets out of bed, comes downstage a bit, and stands attentively. Biff is two years older than his brother Happy, well built, but in these days bears a worn air and seems less self-assured. He has succeeded less, and his dreams are stronger and less acceptable than Happy's. Happy is tall, powerfully made. Sexuality is like a visible color on him, or a scent that many women have discovered. He, like his brother, is lost, but in a different way, for he has never allowed himself to turn his face toward defeat and is thus more confused and hard-skinned, although seemingly more content.)* (p. 11)

> *(Charley has appeared in the doorway. He is a large man, slow of speech, laconic, immovable. In all he says, despite what he says, there is pity, and, now, trepidation. He has a robe over pajamas, slippers on his feet. He enters the kitchen.)* (p. 29)

Activity

These descriptions given by Miller provide important help for the actors. He is speaking directly to them and to the director about how he sees the characters, and using something like a novelist's technique for the reader's benefit as well. Now that you have read the play right through once, consider how far these descriptions are borne out by the way the characters behave.
Work with a partner to accumulate some evidence of the personality traits suggested in the stage directions, concentrating initially on the first section of the play.

Linda: What evidence can you find in Act I of Linda's devotion to her husband? Find a couple of lines that seem to sum up her "more than love" for him (e.g. p. 25 or p. 39).

Biff and Happy: a) Where in the early scenes can you find evidence of Biff's dreams? Have a look at p. 14 and select a line or two.
b) Find some indication of Happy's "sexuality" in his conversation with Biff in the bedroom (pp. 15–16). Then try to find evidence of his refusal to turn his face towards defeat.

Charley: There are hints here that he feels compassion for Willy; on the next page he even offers him a job. (The offer is refused rather churlishly.) Can you remember any other events later in the play which confirm this impression?

Make brief notes on all these points to use later in work on characters and relationships.

Follow-up

Notice that Willy is not revealed to us in this way, by means of stage directions. His first entrance just shows us his heavy suitcases and his exhaustion; the rest we have to find out gradually from his speech and behaviour.

Start looking at this by examining his first conversation with Linda, pp. 6–11, and note down what evidence you can find of the stress he is under and the beginnings of his disintegration.

Impulse

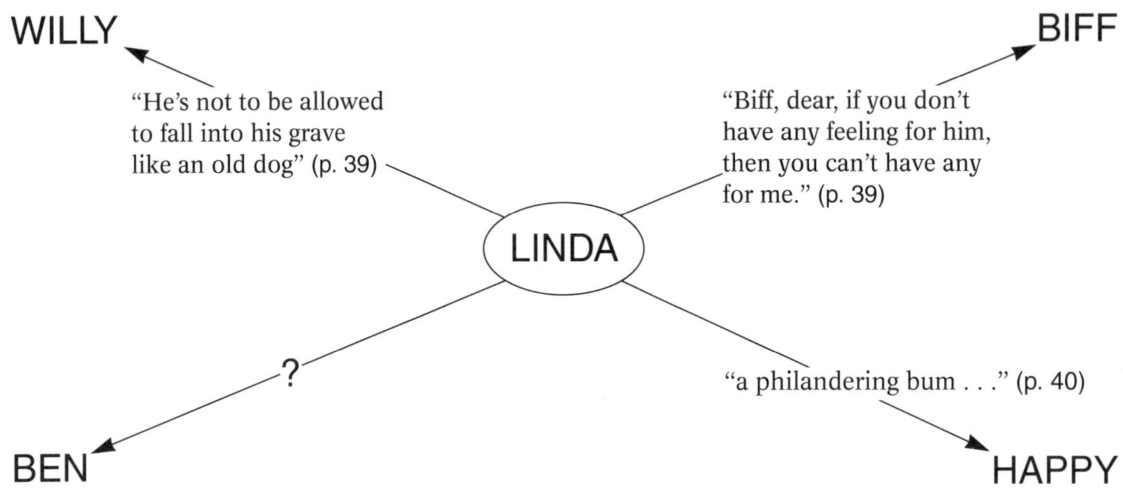

Activity

This is a simple and thought-provoking way of presenting some of the evidence about family relationships you have found in the early sections of the play. You will see that Linda's feelings in Act I are represented by quotations which sum up what she thinks about her husband and her sons. Would you have chosen the same lines? Discuss with a partner what you would have chosen.

When she meets Ben in the first of the memory scenes (pp. 31–36), what does she feel about him? Choose one line to insert in the relevant space in the diagram.

Now copy the diagram again, this time with the arrows pointing in the opposite direction, and consider what each of the characters thinks and feels about Linda. Working with a partner, select one line to crystallize each relationship. Of course this method over-simplifies; the relationships are far too complex to be summed up in this way, but the exercise of thinking and selecting is a valuable one.

Follow-up

The relationship between Linda and Willy is perhaps the most complex of all. Look back over Act I and see what you can find to show how they feel about each other.
Look especially at her defence of him to their sons and at her flattery of him ("You are, Willy. The handsomest man." p. 27).
On his side there is the appearance of The Woman on p. 26, which is not fully explained until later, in Act II, and the symbolism of the stockings, p. 27. He also tells her, "You're the best there is, Linda, you're a pal, you know that?"
When you have collected evidence from Act I, use this as a starting point for a discussion on the following questions:
To what extent does Linda contribute to Willy's situation? Does she help him to escape the truth rather than face up to it? Why does he need The Woman? (And why is she nameless at this point?)

Alternatively, you could choose a volunteer to play Linda and ask her questions to answer in rôle. Discuss her answers and whether they are justified by the evidence in the play so far.

Impulse

In *Timebends,* Miller says:

> "A play ... could cut through time like a knife through a layer cake or a road through a mountain revealing its geological layers, and instead of one incident in one time frame succeeding another, display past and present concurrently, with neither one ever coming to a stop" (p. 131).

It can be useful to sort out the structure of the play in your own mind by presenting the development of the scenes diagrammatically, like this:

Act I
Present — **Past**

p. 6 ff. Willy's return; conversation with Linda; his confusion apparent.

p. 11 ff. Conversation between boys. Background information and their present position.

Transition: W talking to himself.

pp. 18 ff. First memory scene. Boys when young. Contrast Bernard.

pp. 28 ff. Happy comes down, Charley arrives. Card game.

Confusion of past and present.

Ben arrives.
pp. 34 ff. Ben talks about father, meets boys. Building site thefts.

pp. 36 ff. Linda comes down. Tells B and H of W's attempts at suicide.

pp. 44 ff. W returns. Idea of "The Loman Brothers, Sporting Goods".

Activity

Your task is to do the same analysis for Act II. This will be more complicated because of the greater number of memory scenes, but it is worth doing in order to gain a clear picture of the structure of the play.

Follow-up

1. One of the ways in which Miller helps the audience to know whether the action at any point is in present or past is by means of the setting. In Unit 5 we examined the way the actors are told to use the setting differently in past and present, and there are other, even more obvious, transformations. Do you remember the threatening apartment houses of the opening? Look at this stage direction from p. 18:
   "The apartment houses are fading out and the entire house and surroundings become covered with leaves. Music insinuates itself as the leaves appear."

   This marks the beginning of the first memory scene, and almost every time we move into the past the setting changes in this way.

   Take time to skim through the whole play and note down the changes of setting in this way and pages where they occur. Mark them in some way on your chart.

2. You will also have noticed that there are some occasions when past and present are mixed up in Willy's mind, as when Ben arrives while Willy and Charley are playing cards (p. 31), and when The Woman appears (p. 26). Look also at the restaurant scene in Act II, where Willy's memories and his conversation with Biff are very confused, and the end of the second act (p. 97), when Ben seems to take on a different function and become the other half of Willy's mind rather than a memory.

   Mark all these examples, and any others you find, on your chart.

UNIT 9 Contrasts and parallels

Impulse

Look at these two extracts:

BERNARD: Biff! [He *gets away from* HAPPY.] Listen Biff, I heard Mr Birnbaum say that if you don't start studyin' math he's gonna flunk you, and you won't graduate. I heard him!
WILLY: You better study with him, Biff. Go ahead now.
BERNARD: I heard him!
BIFF: Oh, Pop, you didn't see my sneakers! [*He holds up a foot for* WILLY *to look at.*]
WILLY: Hey, that's a beautiful job of printing!
BERNARD [*wiping his glasses*]: Just because he printed University of Virginia on his sneakers doesn't mean they've got to graduate him, Uncle Willy!
WILLY [*angrily*]: What're you talking about? With scholarships to three universities they're gonna flunk him?
BERNARD: But I heard Mr Birnbaum say –
WILLY: Don't be a pest, Bernard! [*To his boys*] What an anaemic!

p. 22

CHARLEY [*an arm on* bernard's *shoulder*]: How do you like this kid? Gonna argue a case in front of the Supreme Court.
BERNARD [*protesting*]: Pop!
WILLY [*genuinely shocked, pained, and happy*]: No! The Supreme Court!
BERNARD: I gotta run. 'Bye, Dad!
CHARLEY: Knock 'em dead, Bernard!
[BERNARD *goes off.*]
WILLY [*as* CHARLEY *takes out his wallet*]: The Supreme Court! And he didn't even mention it!
CHARLEY [*counting out money on the desk*]: He don't have to – he's gonna do it.
willy: And you never told him what to do, did you? Your never took any interest in him.
charley: My salvation is that I never took any interest in anything.

pp. 68–69

There's a great sense of irony here, isn't there? Bernard, the 'anaemic', who hero-worshipped Biff, has become the successful one, in both intellectual and social terms, while Biff has failed in every job, been to jail and never managed to "find himself". In the earlier part of the scene we also find out that Bernard is married, with two boys of his own. Biff depends on his brother's pickups for a good time. The contrast between them brings out very clearly the frustration of Biff, and Willy's failure to bring up his boys with any proper moral standards. Even Willy is struck by the contrast; hence his question to Bernard, "What's . . . the secret?" (p. 66).

Activity

Work in groups of four or five. In each group, choose one student to become Bernard as an adult. Ask him for his version of events, and he tries to answer your questions in rôle. Before you begin, have another look at the scene in Charley's office, pp. 65 – 68.

What would Bernard remember about Biff and his feelings for him? (Remember he begged to be allowed to carry some of the equipment for the Ebbets Field game.) Why did he help Biff so much with his studies? What did he think about Biff's refusal to go back for Summer School? Some of these are answered in the script, but others will require you to use your imagination.

Discuss the answers your "Bernard" gives, and don't be afraid to disagree if you think the character would give different answers.

Follow-up

Examine some of the other contrasts and parallels that exist in the play. Work with a partner to write down points in columns to bring out the contrasts and similarities between the following:

Willy's and Biff's relationship/
Charley's and Bernard's relationship

Howard as a businessman/
Charley as a businessman

Ben's success/
Willy's professional failure

Willy and women/
Happy and women

Display your lists to the rest of the class and discuss them.

UNIT 10 Character jigsaw: Happy

Impulse

Look again at the following extracts.

HAPPY [*moving about with energy, expressiveness*]: All I can do now is wait for the merchandise manager to die. And suppose I get to be merchandise manager? He's a good friend of mine, and he just built a terrific estate on Long Island. And he lived there about two months and sold it, and now he's building another one. He can't enjoy it once it's finished. And I know that's just what I would do. I don't know what the hell I'm workin' for. Sometimes I sit in my apartment – all alone. And I think of the rent I'm paying. And it's crazy. But then, it's what I always wanted. My own apartment, a car, and plenty of women. And still, goddammit, I'm lonely.

HAPPY: Sure, the guy's in line for the vice-presidency of the store. I don't know what gets into me, maybe I just have an over-developed sense of competition or something, but I went and ruined her, and furthermore I can't get rid of her. And he's the third executive I've done that to. Isn't that a crummy characteristic? And to top it all, I go to their weddings!

HAPPY [*grabbing* BIFF, *shouts*]: Wait a minute! I got an idea. I got a feasible idea. Come here, Biff, let's talk this over now, let's talk some sense here. When I was down in Florida last time, I thought of a great idea to sell sporting goods. It just came back to me. You and I, Biff – we have a line, the Loman Line. We train a couple of weeks, and put on a couple of exhibitions, see?
WILLY: That's an idea!
HAPPY: Wait! We form two basketball teams, see? Two water-polo teams. We play each other. It's a million dollars worth of publicity. Two brothers, see? The Loman Brothers. Displays in the Royal Palms – all the hotels. And banners over the ring and the basketball court: "Loman Brothers".

HAPPY: I'm gonna get married, Mom. I wanted to tell you.
LINDA: Go to sleep, dear.
HAPPY [*going*]: I just wanted to tell you.
WILLY: Keep up the good work. [HAPPY *exits*.]

Activity

Read through these extracts aloud with a partner, taking it in turns to be Happy, and discuss what picture of the character they create. These examples are all from Act I.

Now look up the following passages from Act II and select a line or two to sum up each of them:

1. The section of the Restaurant Scene where Happy "chats up" the Girl (pp. 72–74), and especially the boasts (quite false, of course) about West Point and Biff's football prowess.
2. His view that Biff would be crazy to tell his father the truth about the disastrous visit to Bill Oliver (pp. 7 –76).
3. The line, "No, that's not my father. He's just a guy." (p. 84) What does it reveal about Happy?
4. His reassertion of Willy's values in the Requiem, p. 102 ll. 14–15: "He had a good dream . . . "

Now you have collected a whole range of quotations spoken by Happy, representing different aspects of his character. Your task is to create and present a picture of his personality, using some of these lines. Work in groups of four or five and devise your presentation of "the essential Happy Loman". Put the lines in any order you like – you could start with the Requiem if you wish, allowing the others to appear out of the past, or show Happy as a boy followed by Happy as a man, if you prefer.
Try to use movement, too, to increase the drama of your picture of him: the speakers of the lines could circle round him, bombarding him with his own thoughts. Try to ensure that everyone in the group takes part in some way.

Follow-up

Howard

Howard only appears in one scene, but there is quite a lot of evidence of his character here. Read through the scene (pp. 54–60) and select some lines which show his character clearly. Now pool your ideas with the rest of your group and use some of the lines to put together a 'jigsaw' picture of Howard.

Here are some of the things you will need to include:
His feeling that his new 'toy' is more important than Willy; his reaction to Willy's request for a New York job; his reactions to Willy's emphasis on the past; his callous request that Willy "stop by and drop off the samples"; his embarrassment at Willy's emotion.

Weave these into a composite presentation, just as you did with Happy.

UNIT 11 Auditions

Impulse

Look carefully at the following passages and think about what aspects of Charley's character each of them represents:

1. pp. 29–32 (the card game, up to Charley's exit): What does Willy despise about him? What is his attitude to Willy?
2. p. 35 (Charley warns Willy about his sons' stealing from the building site): What does this tell us about him?
3. pp. 63–64 (before Biff plays at Ebbets Field): Notice how he teases Willy about the Ebbets Field Game by pretending he has forgotten all about it.
4. pp. 69–71 (in the reception room of Charley's office): What help does he offer Willy in this scene?
5. pp. 101–102 (the Requiem): What can we learn of him from his comments on Willy's way of life?

Activity

Work in pairs. From all the material you have examined, choose *three* short extracts that seem to you most indicative of Charley's character. These are to be used by the "casting director" as audition pieces.

Join with another pair and let them audition using your selected pieces. You can then try theirs. In each case, don't just offer the "actors" the passages "cold" but guide them, showing them what you want them to get out of the lines. The pieces can be speeches or dialogue.

Follow-up

Discuss within your group (the two pairs) what kind of performance the part of Charley demands. What should he look like? What kind of a voice should he have? Should he laugh a lot? How would he behave towards his son, Bernard? If you think that he has warmth, how can an actor show this (through gestures, e.g. touching people?).

Now, individually, write up your "Director's Notes" for the actor who is to play Charley in your imaginary production. Point out any aspects or particular sections of the play that seem to you particularly significant and helpful in establishing the character.

UNIT 12 A change of perspective: Linda

Impulse

LINDA: Is this Ben?
BEN [*gallantly*]: How do you do, my dear?
LINDA: Where've you been all these years? Willy's always wondered why you –
WILLY [*pulling* BEN *away from her impatiently*]: Where is Dad? Didn't you follow him? How did you get started?
BEN: Well, I don't know how much you remember.
WILLY: Well, I was just a baby, of course, only three or four years old –
BEN: Three years and eleven months.
WILLY: What a memory, Ben!
BEN: I have many enterprises, William, and I have never kept books.
WILLY: I remember I was sitting under the wagon in – was it Nebraska?
BEN: It was South Dakota, and I gave you a bunch of wild flowers.
WILLY: I remember you walking away down some open road.
BEN: [*laughing*]: I was going to find Father in Alaska.
WILLY: Where is he?
BEN: At that age I had a very faulty view of geography, William. I discovered after a few days that I was heading due south, so instead of Alaska, I ended up in Africa.
LINDA: Africa!
WILLY: The Gold Coast!
BEN: Principally diamond mines.
LINDA: Diamond mines!
BEN: Yes, my dear. But I've only a few minutes –

This is Willy's memory of Linda's first meeting with his brother Ben. He sees Ben as a bold adventurer whose way of life is attractive, and he tries to impress him with talk of "hunting" in Brooklyn etc (p. 35). There are some hints, however, that Linda doesn't quite share his view of Ben; even in Willy's version of events she shows alarm at Ben's behaviour towards Biff (p. 34, when Ben challenges Biff to fight).

Activity

Try to imagine what Linda's memory of this meeting would be and write it in diary form, recording her impressions of Ben at the time.

A second encounter between Linda and Ben is depicted in the play, as seen through Willy's eyes (pp. 60–62, where Ben offers Willy a chance to join him in Alaska). Again it is clear that Linda sees things differently. Add Linda's impressions of this second meeting to her "diary".

We never meet Ben in the scenes of the present; in fact, he has recently died, as Willy tells Charley (p. 31). This means that we see Ben solely as Willy sees him in his memories.

Follow-up

Charley's viewpoint

Look again at Unit 11 and the analysis of Charley. Imagine that as he leaves the funeral he looks back on the events that led to Willy's death. Use his speech about being a salesman (pp. 101–102) as a starting-point and continue it as a flow of thoughts, a kind of interior monologue, to show what he is feeling about Willy's life.

Perhaps he might begin with something like "I realized something serious had started to go wrong that night when I wandered round to see why he was up so late . . .".

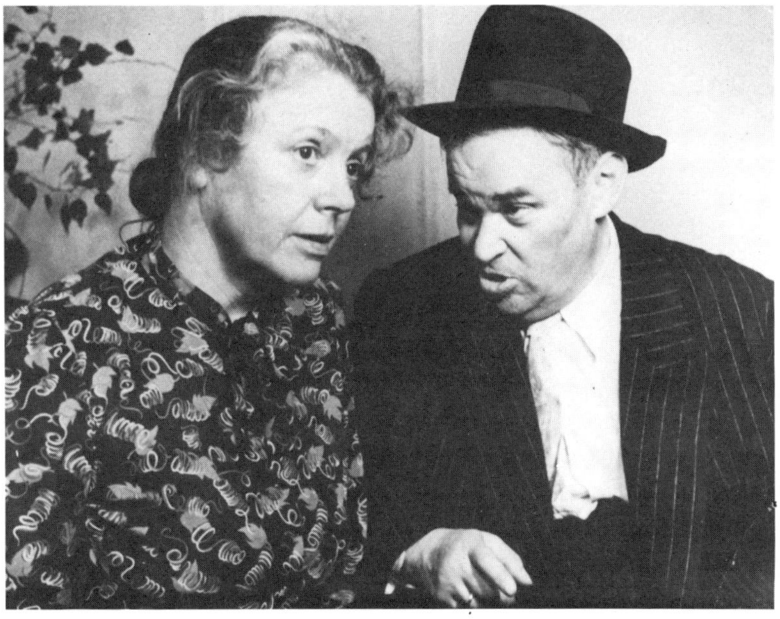

Johanna Hofer as Linda and Fritz Kostner as Willy in a German production of the play (Hebbel-Theater Berlin, 1950)

UNIT 13 Ben and the great outdoors

Impulse

WILLY: No, Ben, I don't want you to think . . . [*He takes* BEN's *arm to show him.*] It's Brooklyn, I know, but we hunt too.
BEN: Really, now.
WILLY: Oh, sure, there's snakes and rabbits and – that's why I moved out here. Why, Biff can fell any one of these trees in no time! Boys! Go right over to where they're building the apartment house and get some sand. We're gonna rebuild the entire front stoop right now! Watch this, Ben!
BIFF: Yes, sir! On the double, Hap!

Ben only exists in Willy's memory. In other words, we cannot be sure the picture we are given of him has much to do with reality. In fact, it's very hard to believe in anyone who has such a faulty view of geography that he sets out for Alaska and ends up in Africa; there must be an element of caricature about Ben. To Willy he represents a link with the romance of the pioneering America of his childhood and earlier; he sees him as a daring heroic figure. Look at the scene where Ben invites Willy to join him in Alaska (pp. 60–61). Do you think that without Linda's objections Willy might have agreed to go? Or was it always only a dream? He has already tried to impress Ben with tales of hunting in Brooklyn and sent the boys off to steal wood to prove their "fearlessness" (see above).

Activity

Look up the following passages in the play.

1. p. 22 (Bernard urges Biff to study for Math): What does Willy call Bernard, and what does this show us of his view of what an American boy should be? (Later he reproaches Bernard for not giving Biff the answers in the Math exam – ironic, isn't it?)
2. p. 31 (Ben's appearance during the card game): What does Willy despise about Charley? Look also at Willy's ability to work with his hands as expressed by Biff and Charley in the Requiem, p. 101.
3. Notice how eager he is to hear about the wild and romantic life of his father from Ben (p. 34).
4. Finally, consider the seed-planting near the end (p. 91). We have already heard that nothing will grow there because of the apartment houses and that Willy has tried before, but he is determined to try one last time. What symbolic meaning could this seed-planting have, do you think?

Join in groups of four or five and discuss what you can learn about Willy from these indicators, and also what it is that he so much admires in Brother Ben. Why should it be his advice that Willy seeks about the suicide and insurance? Now choose someone to be Ben, to answer your questions in rôle. He should try to convey his values ("Never fight fair with a stranger, boy!" etc) and show how they differ from Willy's.

Ben represents another, and almost contradictory, side of the American Dream – the rugged, self-reliant pioneer who goes in covered waggon to the West – or, as in this case, to Alaska. To many Americans the pioneer is a kind of folk-hero such as those celebrated in countless Western films.

Do you think Willy could have been happier if he had not been a salesman? If perhaps he *had* gone with Ben to Alaska? Would a life of adventure have satisfied some need in his nature?

Follow-up

Willy and Linda both try to convince Ben that Willy is a success. It would be useful to compare the two sides of Willy's character – the practical man and the salesman. Use two columns to present these two aspects:

Practical and active	Salesman
Puts up ceiling Admires sporting ability in Biff "I got so many fine tools" (Act II, p. 51)	Needs to be liked Laughed at Loses job

This is only a beginning. Add your own points.

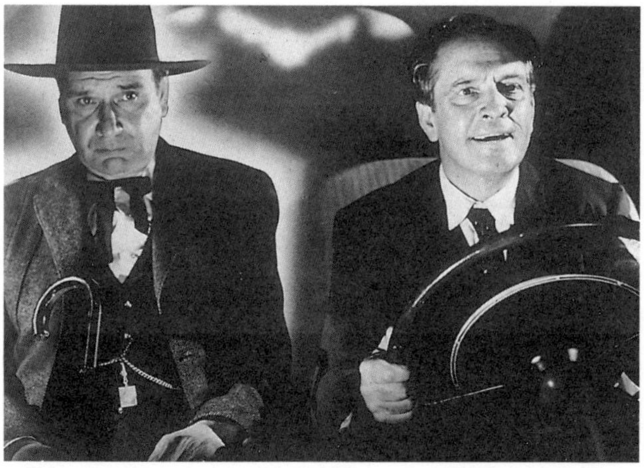

"Ben" and "Willy", 1951

Impulse

More than three-quarters of the play is over before the audience finds out for certain what has been souring the relationship between Biff and his father for so long. (See also Unit 16 *Spotlight on Biff.*)

Look again at the hotel scene, where The Woman suddenly appears (p. 86 l. 1– p. 87 l. 51).
This event from the past, remembered by Willy, is seen to have many repercussions; in fact we become aware of many of them before we understand what caused them. Picture this scene in Boston as a pebble dropped into water, with ripples representing its many consequences.

Activity

Devise a *ripple chart* (see below) to show these results, or some of them. Biff refuses summer school as a direct outcome of the experience, but more follows from this. Didn't it also lead to his leaving home? And perhaps even to his taking to crime? And what about the effects on Willy? (Does his anger at Linda darning her stockings show us anything?)

Follow-up

Turn now to the end of the play. What are the results of Willy's death likely to be? Has anyone or anything really changed?

You can work this out on another diagram if you wish, or just make notes on what you feel will be different or the same – for a class discussion.

Do you find any evidence that Happy is going to become yet another version of his father?

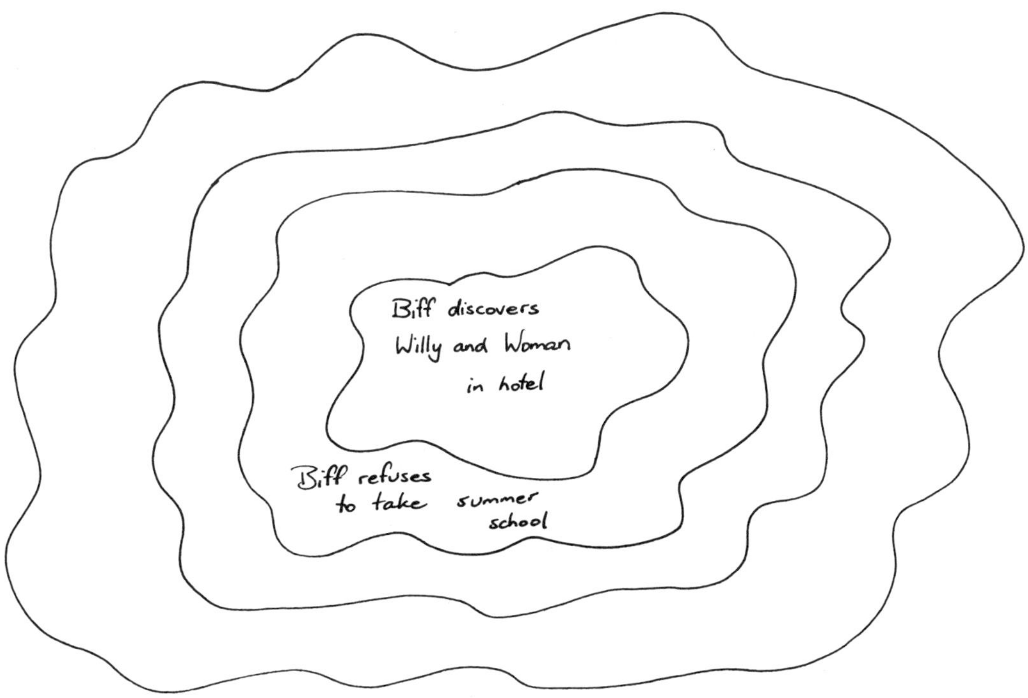

Impulse

Apart from the Loman family and Willy's brother, Ben, we are shown a number of lesser characters, some of them important to the plot or the theme, some of quite minor importance:

The Woman
Howard
Miss Forsythe and Letta
Charley
Bernard
Stanley, the waiter
Jenny, Charley's secretary

Think about each of these and try to decide what is the main function of each in the play. Discuss your views with the students around you.

Activity

Complete the chart below to show what you think is important about each of the minor characters.

For instance:

Character / **Function**	Contrasts with another character	Reveals aspect of another character	Adds humour	Useful to plot; furthers action			**Function explained**
Charley	√		√				Contrast: Howard.
Bernard	√	√					Contrast: Biff. Shows Biff cheating.
The Woman		√					
Howard							
Letta & Miss Forsythe							
Stanley							
Jenny							

Fill in the chart, adding anything else you can think of and completing the list of characters.

Follow-up

Imagine you are one of the least important characters in the play who has very little to say but is in a position to observe at least one piece of the action.
Now write your character's diary, recording the events you have witnessed and your reactions to them. (Letta or Miss Forsythe perhaps? or Stanley?)

or
Improvise the scene of the character returning home and reporting on what he/she has seen and heard. (Howard could tell his wife of the interview with Willy or The Woman could tell a friend all about the meeting with Biff in the Boston hotel room.)

UNIT 16 Spotlight on Biff

Impulse

BIFF [*his weeping breaking from him*]: Dad . . .
WILLY [*infected by it*]: Oh, my boy . . .
BIFF: Dad . . .
WILLY: She's nothing to me, Biff. I was lonely, I was terribly lonely.
BIFF: You – You gave her Mama's stockings! [*His tears break through and he rises to go.*]
WILLY [*grabbing for* BIFF]: I gave you an order!
BIFF: Don't touch me, you – liar!
WILLY: Apologise for that!
BIFF: You fake! You phony little fake! You fake! [*Overcome, he turns quickly and weeping fully goes out with his suitcase.* WILLY *is left on the floor on his knees.*]
WILLY: I gave you an order! Biff, come back here or I'll beat you! Come back here! I'll whip you! (Act II, pp. 87–88)

Biff's exit from the Boston hotel room marks the breakdown of the close relationship between Willy and his elder son. Look over the scene to remind yourself of what happens.

This is the first time the audience is fully aware of the reason for this breakdown, but it is certainly not the first hint that there is trouble between them. Look at Willy's words about him to Linda (p. 8) and at Linda's questioning of Biff (p. 41: "What happened to the love you had for him? You were such pals . . ."). There is another clue (pp. 41–42) when Biff thinks Linda's comment about "a woman" refers to the one in Boston. We also see Willy remembering The Woman (pp. 26–27), but we don't know for certain what has caused the rift until the Boston hotel scene.

Activity

You are going to put together all the evidence you can find about Biff's life story. Much of this has occurred before the play opens, of course, and a good deal will have to come from Willy's memories, which may be unreliable. Nevertheless we can find out quite a lot about Biff.

Each of you adopts one of the roles listed below (or perhaps another). It will be better to work in groups, with each of the characters represented once in each group. The aim is for each of you to present a part of Biff's story, from the point of view of the character you are representing, as if for a television programme (e.g. "This is your life" or "Spotlight on Biff Loman"). The portrait presented by your group should be as comprehensive as possible.

First of all, find out all the relevant situations in the play in which "your" character could have gained some impression of Biff. Then work out what you will say about Biff in the programme.

The "witnesses":

These are only suggestions. You may wish to add some other characters invented on the evidence found in the play (e.g. the coach).

A couple of notes are included alongside "Happy" to give you the idea.

1. HAPPY – Biff's reputation at high school, Biff's ambitions; the changes in Biff; the restaurant scene . . .
2. BERNARD
3. THE COACH – the borrowed football . . .
4. UNCLE BEN
5. CHARLEY
6. WILLY
7. THE WOMAN
8. BIFF HIMSELF
9. LINDA
10. BILL OLIVER – the basket balls? the fountain pen?
11. MISS FORSYTHE

In each group you will need a host for your programme, a moderator who will ask the right questions to encourage each "witness" to tell his or her story about Biff.

Follow-up

This exercise stops short just before Willy's death. In the light of all the evidence you have heard, as well as the feelings Biff himself expresses in the last scenes of the play, write an essay on how Biff has changed by the time of the funeral. Has he learnt anything important? Would he regret anything? What are the chances of a happy and fulfilling life for him, do you think?

You could approach this as a formal essay, remembering that evidence must be confined to what the play actually tells us – or you could write it as Biff's own thoughts as he looks back, in his own voice.

UNIT 17 Hot seat

Impulse

Several times in earlier units you have been asked to volunteer to answer questions in rôle as one of the play's characters. This unit goes a step further in the same direction.

First of all, read again the whole of the Requiem to remind yourselves of the feelings of Charley, Biff, Happy and Linda when the play ends.

Remind yourself also of Howard's attitude to business by looking back at the work you did for Unit 10 (Follow-up).

Activity

Work in groups of about six and allocate one of each of the following characters to each student:

Willy
Linda
Biff
Happy
Charley
Howard

Sit in a semi-circle with a chair facing you. This is the "Hot Seat", and when sitting on it you must answer in rôle. The rest of the students, out of rôle for the time being, ask questions. You will find that motives and relationships offer the most rewarding field.

You might ask Willy:	"Why did you encourage your boys to steal from the building site?"
or Charley:	"Why did you continue to help Willy when he was so churlish and ungrateful?"
or Howard:	"Did you not feel any sense of loyalty to such a long-serving member of your staff as Willy Loman?"

Follow-up

Choose any character you have not examined closely up to now and record his/her feelings at a specified point in the action, as a stream of thoughts.

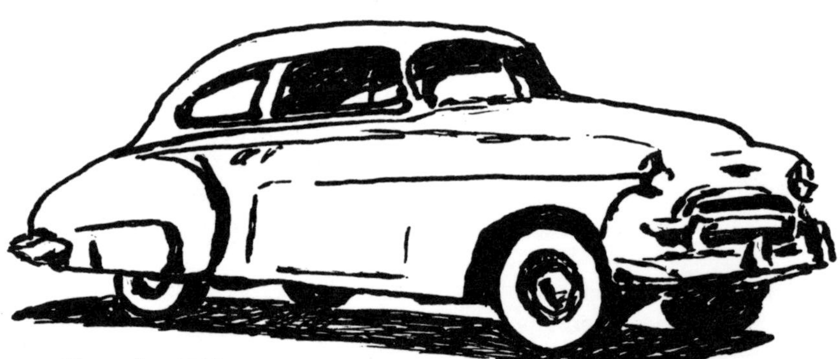

Chevrolet, 1949

Impulse

There can be few plays in which the method of staging is more important and more specifically directed by the dramatist than *Death of a Salesman*.

> "I had known all along that this play could not be encompassed by conventional realism, and for one integral reason: in Willy the past was as alive as what was happening at the moment, sometimes even crashing in to completely overwhelm his mind. I wanted precisely the same fluidity in the form, and now it was clear to me that this must be primarily verbal." (*Timebends*, p. 182).

Miller was searching for a new form that would allow him to present the "inside" of a character's head. In the Preface to his *Collected Plays* he tells us how he first thought of the play:

> "The first image that occurred to me which was to result in *Death of a Salesman* was an enormous face to the height of the proscenium arch which would appear and then open up, and we would see the inside of a man's head. In fact, **The Inside of His Head** was the first title."

In *Timebends,* Miller explains what this meant in terms of the plot. He was, he says, aiming at

> "... an arched flow of storytelling with neither transitional dialogue nor a single fixed locale, a mode that would open a man's head for a play to take place inside it, evolving through concurrent rather than consecutive actions" (*Timebends*, p. 129).

The structure of the play as it evolved in writing was the mixture of past and present in Willy's memory scenes. (This is somewhat akin to, though not identical with, the model of "flashback" in the cinema.) These scenes from the past are interspersed with contrasting scenes of the present (see Unit 8). Such a complex structure required careful staging: set design, lighting and sound are all used to help the audience to know when and where they are at any given point. Sometimes past and present are confused, as in the card-playing scene in Act I, when Ben arrives (pp. 31–32), and in the restaurant in Act II, but it is always important for the audience to distinguish past from present.

Stage directions are very specific in this play, as when Miller explains at the beginning how the set is to be treated differently by the actors in scenes from the past (p. 5 ll. 23–25). See also Unit 5.

Activity

Work in small groups. Divide up the play between you so that each of you examines a particular section to see what role is played by *lighting* and *sound*, e.g.

1. *Lighting*
– in the transition to the first memory scene, where the apartment houses become trees (p. 18);
– during, and after, Willy's reminiscences at the end of Act I (p. 49).
In many other places changes in lighting are implied rather than specific, as in transitions from the house to Howard's office etc.
The Woman behind the scrim (p. 26) also requires lighting effects.
Think about the end of the play and what is demanded of lighting in the transition to the Requiem etc.

2. *Sound*
– music at the opening of the play;
– music when Ben tells Willy about their father (p. 34);
– "bright music" at the beginning of Act II (p. 50).

Collect as many other examples as you can and discuss the effect that is intended in each case.

Follow-up

When you have looked at all these examples of how technical devices are used by Miller, choose a particular section of the play, of about four or five pages, and work as a team to design a setting, drawing up a list of cues for lighting and sound. Try to remain true to Miller's intentions, but do not be afraid to use your own ideas, too. The best way to present your plans might be to photocopy the section and write instructions to the stage crew on the right hand side, opposite the relevant lines. A set plan or sketch should accompany your stage management notes.

Impulse

As we have discovered, there is more to this play than realism. The lighting devices and the use of music, especially the flute music, take on more than surface reality and become symbolic of underlying themes and feelings. We are told that the flute music speaks of "grass and trees and the horizon" (p. 5), but there are other symbolic elements that are left for us to interpret, such as the stockings and the seeds.

Activity

Divide into small groups. Pin large pieces of paper – one for each group – to the wall. Half of the groups are to look for quotes related to the *stockings*, the others for quotes concerning the *seeds* Willy plants, plus related references to the garden. (You could divide the play into segments within your group, with each person searching for quotes in one segment only.)
Write your "symbol" in the middle of your sheet of paper.

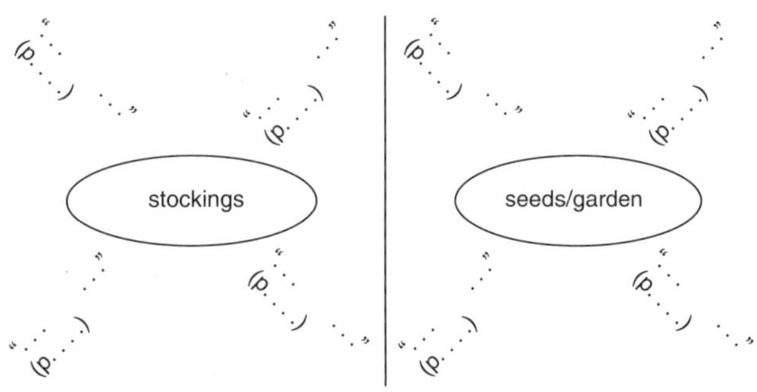

Around your symbol, group the quotes you find, with page numbers. When you have finished, discuss your findings as a class; remember that the *context* of each quote is important.
What do the stockings mean to Willy? To The Woman? To Linda? To the audience?
What do the seeds mean to Willy and the audience?

Follow-up

Take down the essence of your findings and your discussion in note form.

You will no doubt be able to think of other examples of symbolism (are Ben's diamonds in the jungle real or symbolic?). Use your ideas as the basis of a discussion in small groups of three or four.

Then, thinking of all the images that seem to you symbolic of the play, imagine you are the publicity team for a production of the play. Sketch designs for posters, handbills and a programme cover. Some of you might prefer to write a press hand-out about the imaginary production, or the programme notes.

Look at the design of this handbill. What do you think it is intended to convey about the play? What images does the director want to plant in the audience's mind before seeing the play?

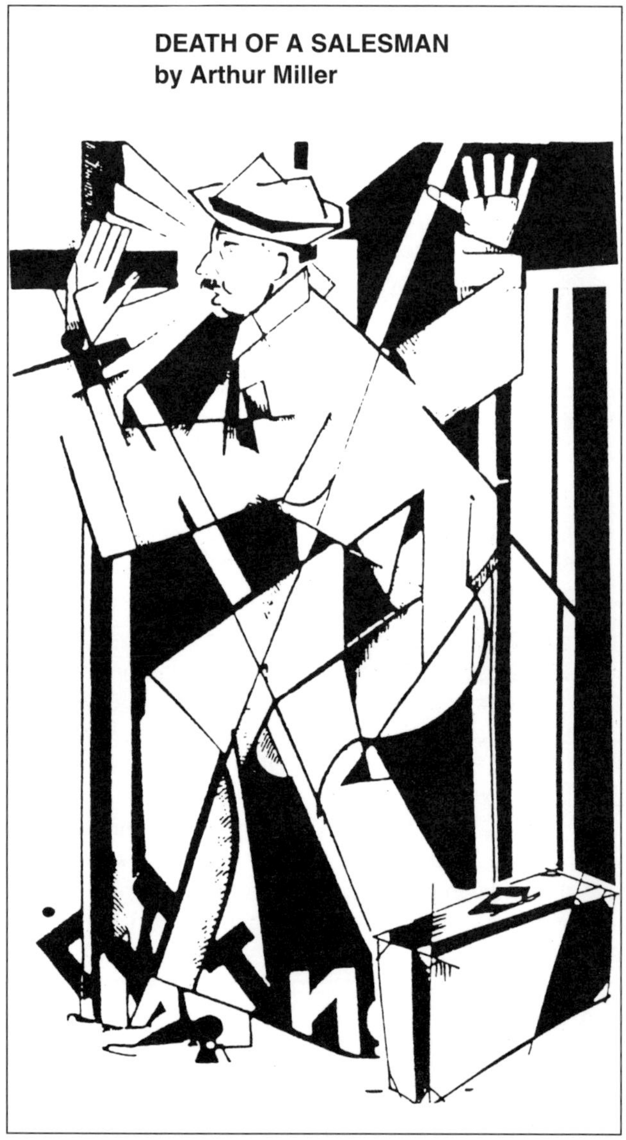

Display your own work for the rest of the class to see.

UNIT 20 The salesman

Impulse

Read once more what Charley says about the profession of Salesman in the Requiem (pp. 101–102).

Now look back at the earlier units which dealt with the themes of success and the American Dream (Units 1 and 2) and consider how the values of a materialistic society coloured Willy's ambitions and fears.

Look particularly at the quotation from *Timebends*, in Unit 2, in which the unnamed American woman accuses Miller of putting a "timebomb under American capitalism".

Activity

Make out a case against the "American Dream", forgetting for the moment any part Willy's own personality played in his downfall. Find as much evidence as you can of Miller blaming capitalism and the values of materialism. Notice that Ben is not without similar values, for all his adventuring; he has a similar ruthlessness to Howard's when he tells Biff, "Never fight fair with a stranger, boy . . ." (p. 34).

Use all the material you have collected for a class discussion on:
Miller's views on materialistic society.

Follow-up

Miller was accused of left-wing sympathies by a number of Americans, and the making of the film of *Salesman* brought some of these out into the open. The makers of the film wanted to screen a specially made 'short' in front of it at every showing, with professors of New York City Business School explaining that Willy Loman was not typical and that nowadays selling was a fine profession with both spiritual and financial compensations. Miller's comment was:

> "In fact they all sounded like Willy Loman with a diploma."

He objected strongly to the short and refused to accept it. In the end they gave way, and the film was shown without it.

Miller insists, in *Timebends*, that the play's attack is not solely upon American capitalism; the message is applicable to many countries and cultures. A production in the USSR which caricatured Willy as a complete fool and made Charley a clownish idiot (because as business men they could not have a shred of sincerity!) would seem to bear this out.

A production in China, which Miller himself helped to direct, makes the same point, as he records in *Timebends*:

> Willy was representative everywhere, in every kind of system, of ourselves in this time. The Chinese might disapprove of his lies and his self deluding exaggerations as well as his immorality with women, but they certainly saw themselves in him. And it was not simply as a type but because of what he wanted. Which was to excel, to win out over anonymity and meaninglessness, to love and be loved, and above all perhaps to COUNT . . . "I am not a dime a dozen! I am Willy Loman, and you are Biff Loman!" (*Timebends*, p. 184).

Work in threes to create a TV arts programme in which a chairperson or host directs a discussion between two critics of the very first production of the play. Their views are diametrically opposed. One finds the play "un-American" in its values, the other defends the play's message.

Alternatively, you could work individually to write a letter to the lady who called the play 'a time-bomb under American capitalism', answering her criticisms in any way you choose.

Impulse

LINDA: Then make Charley your father, Biff. You can't do that, can you? I don't say he's a great man. Willy Loman never made a lot of money. His name was never in the paper. He's not the finest character that ever lived. But he's a human being, and a terrible thing is happening to him. So attention must be paid. He's not to be allowed to fall into his grave like an old dog. Attention, attention must be finally paid to such a person. (p. 39)

This moving speech of Linda's does a great deal to win the audience's sympathy for Willy. Yet we do see much in him to blame: he frequently lies, he cheats on his wife, he brings up his sons to steal and to cheat in exams, and to believe that personal attractiveness is all that counts. It is the balance between pity and blame that creates a sense of tragedy, together with the realization, as Linda says, that he is human, like ourselves, and full of very human faults.

Activity

Who or what do you think bears the greatest blame for what happened to Willy? One way of reviewing the whole play is to stage an inquest to establish any blame there may be. There are a number of characters who could be questioned about their part in the tragedy.

Willy himself: Plenty to find here, especially in his self-deception. Of course, we must divorce ourselves from reality here in assuming Willy can speak about his own death.
Linda: She never helps him to face the truth.
Biff: Did his row with his father precipitate the suicide?
Howard: Was his sacking of Willy the last straw?
Ben: Were the dreams of success unsettling, and what about the discussion about the insurance?
Happy: He tries to preserve Willy's illusions. Is this fatal for Willy?

There may be other characters you wish to include, or some of these you feel can be left out. Allocate one person to each role, and the rest become the coroners, asking questions. Take time to look through relevant passages in the play and prepare these questions, or the answers you will give. Then proceed with the inquest. You can draw up your own rules for the proceedings.

After all the witnesses have been questioned, the coroners should discuss their findings in front of the whole group and try to come to some conclusions.

Follow-up

If you have ever seen a tragic play on the stage, you will recognize the special experience it offers an audience, even if you, like many other people over the years, cannot easily define this experience. Look up the term "tragedy" in encyclopaedias and reference books about the theatre, then discuss in pairs what you feel are the essentials. You will probably find most critics emphasize two ingredients:

1. The need to feel that the tragic hero is fully human and yet partly to blame for his own downfall – therefore he must be neither wholly bad (or we will not pity him) nor wholly good (or his downfall will be too painful); and

2. that the ending of the play is never entirely depressing, despite painful disasters.

To what extent do you consider Willy Loman's downfall to be truly tragic? How far is he responsible for his own situation? And how does Miller retain the audience's pity for him? Is there any sense of hope at the end of the play?

This is what William Hawkins wrote of the first production:

> *Death of a Salesman* is a play written along the lines of the finest classical tragedy. It is the revelation of a man's downfall, a destruction whose roots are entirely in his own soul. The play builds to an immutable conflict where there is no resolution for this man in this life.
>
> (William Hawkins, *New York World Telegram*, 11 February 1949)

Do you agree that the roots of Willy's downfall are "entirely in his own soul"?

And perhaps the last word on this should go to Miller himself:

> To me the tragedy of Willy Loman is that he gave his life, or sold it, in order to justify the waste of it. It is the tragedy of a man who did believe that he alone was not meeting the qualifications laid down for mankind by those clean-shaven frontiersmen who inhabit the peaks of broadcasting and advertising offices. From those forests of canned goods high up near the sky, he heard the thundering command to succeed as it ricocheted down the newspaper-lined canyons of his city, heard not a human voice, but a wind of a voice to which no human can reply in kind, except to stare into the mirror at a failure.
>
> (Arthur Miller, *New York Times*, 5 February 1950)

Record your own reactions and opinions on the play as a whole and your conclusions about this 'tragedy', if you see it as one.